Healing the Spirit and Body with Aromatherapy & Essential Oils

Moneva Amanda

Copyright © 2021 Moneva Amanda

All rights reserved. No part of this publication may be reproduced, distributed, or transmitted in any form or by any means, including photocopying, recording, or other electronic or mechanical methods, without the prior written permission of the publisher, except in the case of brief quotations embodied in critical reviews and certain other non-commercial uses permitted by copyright law.

ISBN: 978-1-63750-307-2

Table of Contents

HEALING THE SPIRIT AND BODY WITH AROMATHERAPY, & ESSENTIAL OILS ... 1

PREFACE ... 5

INTRODUCTION ... 7
    How long has aromatherapy been with us? ... 7

CHAPTER 1 ... 9
    HOW DOES AROMATHERAPY TREATMENT WORK? ... 9
    AROMATHERAPY BENEFITS ... 10
        Conditions it can treat ... 11
    POPULAR AROMATHERAPY OILS ... 12

CHAPTER 2 ... 15
    SIDE EFFECTS ... 15

CHAPTER 3 ... 17
    ESSENTIAL OILS AS PAIN RELIEVERS ... 17
        What the studies say ... 18
    ESSENTIAL OILS FOR TREATMENT ... 19
    HOW TO USE ESSENTIAL OILS FOR TREATMENT ... 21
        Dangers and Warnings ... 24

CHAPTER 4 ... 27
    AROMATHERAPY: WHAT YOU SHOULD KNOW ... 27
        Using Aromatherapy ... 28
        Benefits ... 31
    WHAT DO ESSENTIAL OILS DO? ... 33
        Visiting an Aromatherapist ... 36
        Risks ... 37
        Caution when using essential oils ... 38

CHAPTER 5 ... 42

How Aromatherapy Works 42
    The Study on Aromatherapy 42
Ways to use aromatherapy 44
    Topical Use 45
    Side effects and safety 45

CHAPTER 6 47

Essential Oils and Diffusers: The Best Guide 47
    4 Essential Oils for Rest & Relaxation 47
Four essential oils for higher concentration 54
    Four natural oils for emotion & happiness 59
    Warm and Steam Oil Diffusers: How to Use Them 65

CHAPTER 7 69

The Ultimate Essential Oil Guide: the ones to use and for what purpose 69
What Are Essential Oils? 69
What can essential oils be used for? 70
    How should I dilute my natural oils? 71

CHAPTER 8 77

Advantages and Disadvantages of Aromatherapy 77
    Advantages: 77
    Disadvantages: 79
Is aromatherapy right for everybody? 81

CHAPTER 9 85

How to use aromatherapy for stress relief 85
    Research 85
    How to use aromatherapy for stress relieve 87

CHAPTER 10 90

Six most popular new aromatherapy brands 90
    Choosing a Provider 97

Preface

Do you want to feel happier, more creative, and more productive?

Aromatherapy is one of the oldest forms of medicine known to man. It is used today for stress reduction, pain relief and as a natural way to promote good health and a better quality of life. Sometimes it is called oil therapy and it's very effective.

Do you want to be more energetic? Fulfilled? Balanced? Have more energy than you know what to do with?

Did you know that 75% of our immune system is located in our nose? Research shows that the scent of a flower, or essential oil, stimulates the olfactory nerves which is the first line of defense of the immune system. The power of scents in enhancing mood, relieving pain, and promoting relaxation has been known for centuries by many cultures.

When you use essential oils in aromatherapy, you can expect improved physical and emotional energy levels, reduced pain, and a sense of peace and tranquility.

Aromatherapy can even enhance your memory and concentration! To get the maximum benefits from this natural therapy, it should be used consistently, over time. Essential oils are highly concentrated sources of plant chemicals that have potent effects on the mind and body. They can dramatically improve mood, enhance mental performance, and reduce stress. They can also stimulate the lymphatic system, increase circulation, cleanse the skin, and promote healthy hair and nails. You also get to understand aromatherapy recipe for healing the spirit, how to use aromatherapy candle sets for women (including candle making kit), crystal healing for beginners or dummies, oil bath and body works, and effective use of essential oils and healing stones.

Would you like to be more creative, more focused, and less stressed? Aromatherapy can help you achieve these goals. It can also help you lose weight, sleep better, and have more energy! Get some essential oils to start your journey to a healthier, happier you today!

Introduction

Aromatherapy is a holistic healing treatment that uses natural herb extracts to promote health and well-being. Sometimes it is called *oil therapy*. Aromatherapy uses aromatic essential oils medicinally to improve the health of the body, brain, and spirit. It also improves both physical and psychological health.

Aromatherapy is regarded as both a skill and a science. Lately, aromatherapy has gained more recognition in the areas of science and medicine.

How long has aromatherapy been with us?

Humans have used aromatherapy for several years. Old cultures in China, India, Egypt, and other parts of the world included aromatic plant components in resins, balms, and oils. These natural substances were used for medical and spiritual purposes. These were known to have both physical and mental benefits. Essential oils distillation is credited to the Persians in the 10th century, although practice might have been in use for a long time before this period. Information about oil distillation was released in the 16th century in Germany. French doctors in the 19th century acknowledged the potential of essential oils in treating disease.

Doctors became competent in the 19th century and focused on using chemical drugs. However, the French and German doctors still recognized the role of natural botanicals in curing illnesses.

- The word "*aromatherapy*" was coined by a French perfumer and chemist **René-Maurice Gattefossé** in a book he wrote on this topic which was published in 1937. He previously discovered the healing potential of lavender in treating burns.

This book discusses the use of essential oils in treating medical conditions.

CHAPTER 1

How Does Aromatherapy Treatment Work?

Aromatherapy works through the sense of smell and skin absorption using products such as:

- Diffusers

- Aromatic spritzers

- Inhalers

- Bathing salts.

- Body oils, creams, or lotions for therapeutic massage or topical application

- Facial steamers

- Hot and cold compresses

- Clay masks

You might use these alone or in any combination. There are almost a hundred types of essential oils available.

Generally, people use the most popular oils.

Essential oils are available online, in health food stores, and in a few regular supermarkets. It is important to buy a reputable producer because the oils are not regulated by the *FDA*. This helps to ensure that you're buying a good product that is purely natural. It shouldn't contain any additives or synthetic ingredients.

Each essential oil has a selection of unique therapeutic properties, uses, and effects. Combining essential oils to make a synergistic blend creates even more benefits.

Aromatherapy Benefits

Aromatherapy has lots of benefits. It's thought to:

- Manage pain

- Improve rest quality

- Reduce stress, agitation, and anxiety

- Soothe sore joints

- Treat headaches and migraines

- Alleviate side effects of chemotherapy

- Ease discomforts of labor

- Fight bacteria, virus, or fungus

- Improve digestion

- Improve hospice and palliative care

- Boost immunity

Scientific evidence for aromatherapy is known to be limited in some areas. Research to support the use of aromatherapy in treating *Alzheimer's disease, Parkinson's disease, and cardiovascular disease are lacking.*

Conditions it can treat

Aromatherapy has the potential to treat many diseases, such as:

- Asthma

- Insomnia

- Fatigue

- Depression

- Inflammation

- Peripheral neuropathy

- Menstrual issues

- Alopecia

- Cancer

- Erectile dysfunction

- Arthritis

- Menopause

Popular Aromatherapy Oils

According to the National Association for Holistic Aromatherapy, the most popular essential oils are:

- Clary sage

- Cypress

- Eucalyptus
- Fennel
- Geranium
- Ginger
- Helichrysum
- Lavender
- Lemon
- Lemongrass
- Mandarin
- Neroli
- Patchouli
- Peppermint
- Roman chamomile
- Rose
- Rosemary

- Tea tree

- Vetiver

- Ylang

You can use essential oils in several ways. For instance, add them to body lotions or carrier oils. Try improving a cosmetic toner, shampoo, or conditioner with essential oils. Or add them to liquid soap, toothpaste, or mouthwash. You can even diffuse or spritz the oils throughout a room or pour them into a bath.

Chapter 2

Side Effects

Most essential oils are safe to use. But there are a few safety measures you should take when using them, and some side effects you should know about, especially if you take any prescription drugs.

Don't apply essential oils directly to your skin. Always use a carrier oil to dilute the natural oils. Remember to carry out a skin patch test before using essential oils. Since citrus essential natural oils may make your skin more sensitive to sunlight, these natural oils should be avoided if you'll be exposed to sunlight.

Children and women who are pregnant or breastfeeding should use essential oils with caution and under the supervision of a medical doctor. You should avoid some oils and never swallow essential oils.

Side effects of using essential oils include:

- Rashes

- Asthma attacks
- Headaches
- Allergic reactions
- Skin irritation
- Nausea

Use essential oils with caution if you have:

- Hay fever
- Asthma
- Epilepsy
- High blood pressure
- Eczema
- Psoriasis

Chapter 3

Essential oils as pain relievers

If drugs are not easing your pain, you may start thinking of seeking alternative treatment solutions. Essential oils might be one of the natural ways to cure pain.

Essential oils are highly fragrant substances found in the petals, stems, origins, and other parts of plants. They are usually taken off the plant through steam distillation. The oils produced by this centuries-old technique can enhance physical, emotional, and mental wellbeing. Each kind of essential oil has its unique fragrance and benefits. These natural oils can be used separately or as a mix.

Experts have found evidence to claim that certain natural oils may treat the symptoms of certain illnesses, such as:

- Inflammation

- Headaches

- Depression

- Sleep disorders

- Respiratory problems

More research is required to understand how essential natural oils can help to ease pain. Although there is no harm in adding essential natural oils to your pain management plan, and they might enable you to reduce prescriptions doses.

What the studies say

The U.S. Food and Drugs Administration (**FDA**) does not regulate essential oils. This means that essential oil products may differ in purity, power, and quality across manufacturers. Ensure to only buy essential oils from reputable brands.

Essential oils can be inhaled or applied topically when blended with a carrier oil. Never use undiluted essential oils directly on your skin. Also, you should never swallow essential natural oils. Do a skin patch test before using diluted essential oils on your skin.

Essential oils for treatment

- **Lavender**

According to a 2013 research, lavender oil can help to treat pain in children after a tonsillectomy. Children who inhale lavender scent could reduce their daily dose of acetaminophen post-surgery.

Analysts in a 2015 study, discovered that lavender oil can be an effective analgesic and anti-inflammatory. When diluted lavender oil was applied topically during one test, it provided treatments like that of the prescribed drugs tramadol. This shows that lavender can be used to treat pain and any inflammation.

Another study in 2012 tested lavender essential oil's ability to reduce pain in people who experience migraines. Results showed that inhaling the lavender scent was effective in reducing the severity of migraines.

Rose oil

A lot of women experience stomach cramps during menstruation. **Rose oil** aromatherapy has been proven to cure pain related to periods when compared to standard treatment.

A study from 2013 shows that rose oil aromatherapy can also be useful in treating pain caused by kidney stones when used with conventional therapy.

- **Bergamot**

Bergamot oil aromatherapy has been used to treat neuropathic pain, which is often resistant to *opioid pain drugs*. The results of a 2015 study found this treatment to help in reducing *neuropathic pain*.

- **Oil blends**

Researchers in a 2012 research found a blend of essential oils useful in reducing severe and intense menstrual pain. People use lotions made of lavender, clary sage, and marjoram to therapeutically massage their lower abdomen daily.

According to some other study in 2013, an essential oil

blend was successful in reducing discomfort and menstrual blood loss. People were massaged with a blend of cinnamon, clove, and lavender in sweet almond oil. These were massaged once daily for a week before their periods.

Another study showed the potentials of essential oil blends to reduce pain and reduce depression in people who have terminal cancer. These people had their hands massaged with bergamot, lavender, and frankincense in sweet almond oil.

How to use essential oils for treatment

Ensure to use a carrier oil to dilute your preferred oil. Applying undiluted oil can cause skin inflammation and irritation.

Common carrier oils are:

- Coconut
- Avocado
- Sweet almond

- Apricot kernel

- Sesame

- Jojoba

- Grapeseed

In general, you only need to use a few drops of oil. The dose may differ, but a useful recommendation is to add about ten drops of **oil** to every tablespoon of your carrier oil.

Before using a new oil, do a skin patch test to test its effects on your skin. Rub the diluted oil on your forearm. If you don't experience any discomfort or pain within 24 to 48 hours, the oil should be safe for your use.

- **Massage**

Massaging diluted oil on the skin can ease the muscles and relieve pain. You can practice self-massage or decide to consult a professional therapeutic massage using essential oils.

- **Inhalation**

Add a few drops of your preferred oil to a diffuser and inhale the steam in a closed room. No carrier oil is required for this method.

If you don't have a diffuser, you can fill a bath or bowl with warm water. Add a few drops of the oil to the water. Lean on the dish or kitchen sink, cover your head with a towel, and inhale the steam. You can do this for 10 minutes.

- **Hot bath**

You may even take a warm bath with essential oils. To dissolve the essential oil, first, add five drops (*the number of drops may vary based on the kind of oil*) for a drop of carrier oil. If you don't want essential oil in your bath, you can add the drops to a glass of milk, and the oil will blend with the fat in the milk. Sitting in the bath will allow the essential oil to enter your body through the skin. The steam that rises from the warm water can offer extra aromatherapy. *Avoid hot baths, as this can cause weakness or dizziness.*

Dangers and Warnings

Always take extreme care when trying a new essential oil. Take time to dilute essential natural oils in a carrier oil such as olive oil or sweet almond oil. Never apply essential natural oils directly to the skin. Some people can be allergic to some essential oils. To do a patch test, add three to five drops of the natural essential oil with a drop of carrier oil. Apply a little of this mixture to the skin of your forearm, if there is no reaction between 24 to 48 hours, it should be safe for your use.

Consult your doctor before use if you:

- are pregnant

- are nursing

- have a preexisting medical condition

- wish to use essential natural oils on children or old adults

Possible side effects of using essential oils include:

- Skin irritation

- Skin inflammation

- Sun sensitivity

- Allergic reaction

If you'd like to start using essential oils, you need to get your facts straight first by conducting your research. You must understand the basic benefits and dangers associated with each kind of oil.

You also need to buy it from a reputable brand. The **FDA** doesn't regulate essential oils, so the elements in each product may differ across manufacturers. Some essential oils or oil blends may contain added elements that can cause unwanted side effects.

You can buy essential natural oils online or at your neighborhood holistic health store. Besides, it might be helpful to speak with a certified aromatherapist. They can answer any questions you might have, and help you choose from the essential oils suitable for your taste.

Ensure you;

- Always dilute natural oils before applying them to

your skin.

- Do a skin patch test to test for any discomfort or inflammation.

- Avoid applying essential oils on sensitive areas, such as around your eye or near open wounds.

- Discontinue use if you experience any irritation or discomfort.

- Never swallow essential oil.

Chapter 4

Aromatherapy: What you should know

The National Association of Holistic Aromatherapy (*NAHA*) defines aromatherapy as "the therapeutic application or the medicinal use of aromatic substances (*essential oils)* for holistic healing."

In 1997, the International Standards Business (***ISO***) defined essential oil as a "product from plant raw material, either by distillation with water or steam, or from the epicarp of citric fruits through a mechanical process, or by dried distillation."

A lot of essential oils have been found to have various elements of antimicrobial activities and are thought to have antiviral, nematicidal, antifungal, insecticidal, and antioxidant properties. Aromatherapy applications include therapeutic massage, topical applications, and inhalation.

However, users must understand that "natural" products are also chemicals, and they can be harmful if used wrongly. It is recommended to seek the advice of a professional when working with essential oils.

Using Aromatherapy

[Essential Oils]

1. A lot of essential oils can help to increase health and wellness.

2. Aromatherapy is generally used through inhalation or as topical application.

- **Inhalation:** the natural oils evaporate into the air using a diffuser container, aerosol, or essential oil droplets, or inhaled, for example, in a steam bath.

Aside from giving off a pleasant smell, aromatherapy natural oils can provide respiratory disinfection, decongestant, and mental benefits. Inhaling essential oils stimulates the olfactory system, the part of the brain linked to smell, like the nose and the head.

Substances that enter the nose or mouth move to the lungs and through that, to other parts of your body. As the substances reach the brain, they affect the limbic system, which is responsible for emotions, the heartbeat, blood pressure, breathing, long-term memory, stress, and hormone balance. This way, essential oils can have a sensitive yet holistic influence on the body.

- **Topical applications:** massage oils, and bath and skin products are soaked up through the skin. Massaging the area where the essential oil is to be applied can enhance blood circulation and increase absorption. Some claim that some areas that are richer in perspiration glands and hair roots, like the head or hands, may absorb the natural oils more effectively.

Essential oils should never be applied directly to the skin. They need to be diluted with a carrier oil continually. Usually, a few drops of oil for a drop of carrier oil are the guideline. The most common carrier oils are sweet almond oil or olive oil. You are always advised to do an allergies test before trying a new oil.

To do an allergy test:

- Dilute the essential oil in a carrier oil at double the concentration you intend to use

- Rub the blend into a part as big as a quarter in the forearm

- When there is no allergic reaction within 24 to 48 hours, it should be safe for your use.

- Some people complain about developing allergies to essential oils after having used them consistently for a period of time. If a new allergic reaction shows up, such a person should stop using it immediately and avoid its smell.

- To do a 0.5 to at least one 1 percent dilution, use 3 to 6 drops of oil per drop of carrier. For any 5 percent dilution, add 30 drops to 1 ounce of carrier.

- A maximum concentration of 5 percent is usually considered safe for adults.

- Ingesting, or swallowing, essential oils are not

advised. Taken orally, the oils may damage the liver or kidneys.

- They can also result in reactions with other drugs, and they can also cause unexpected damage to the heart.

Benefits

Aromatherapy is a complementary therapy. It generally does not provide a remedy for diseases, rashes, or ailments, but it can support regular treatments of different conditions.

1. Steam bath with essential oil

A eucalyptus steam bath may relieve symptoms of a cold or flu. It has been proven to reduce:

- Nausea

- Pain and body aches

- Stress, agitation, stress, and depression

- Exhaustion and insomnia

- Muscular aches

- Headaches

- Circulatory problems

- Menstrual problems

- Menopausal problems

- Alopecia or hair thinning

Some types of psoriasis could find treatment with aromatherapy, but a doctor should advise about use and treatment plan.

Digestive problems may be eased with peppermint oil, but it should not be swallowed. Teeth ache and mouth sores can be relieved with clove oil, but this, too, should only be used topically rather than swallowed.

Lovers of aromatherapy claim that these and lots of other issues respond well to aromatherapy; however, not all the uses are supported with scientific proof.

What do essential oils do?

Different natural oils have different uses and results. Basil oil is used to improve sight and cure some of the symptoms of depression. It can relieve headaches and migraines. It should be avoided during pregnancy.

Bergamot oil is acclaimed to be beneficial to the urinary system and digestive system. When mixed with eucalyptus oil, it can help to cure skin problems, including those triggered by stress and chickenpox.

2. Rosemary oil

Rosemary oil can soothe the nervous and circulatory systems. Black pepper oil is often used for revitalizing the blood flow, muscle pains and aches, and bruises. Mixed with ginger oil, it is used to reduce arthritis pain and improve versatility.

- *Chamomile oil* can treat eczema

- *Citronella oil* is a member of the lemongrass family and acts as an insect repellent

- *Clove oil* is a topical analgesic, or painkiller, that is often used for toothache. Also, it is used as an antispasmodic antiemetic, to prevent vomiting and nausea, to act as a carminative, stopping oil in the heart. They have antimicrobial, antioxidant, and antifungal properties.

- *Eucalyptus oil* can help to relieve the airways during a cold or flu. It is used with peppermint. Many people are sensitive to eucalyptus, so treatment should be studied.

- *Geranium oil* can be used for skin problems, to reduce stress, as a mosquito repellant.

- *Jasmine oil* is known to be an aphrodisiac. While medical proof is missing, research shows that the smell of jasmine increases beta waves, which are associated with nervousness. Like a stimulant, it can increase penile blood circulation.

- *Lavender oil* can be used as an antiseptic for small cuts and burns and also enhance rest and sleep. It is said to relieve headaches and migraine symptoms.

- *Lemon oil* is known to improve emotions and also to help relieve the symptoms of stress and depression.

- *Rosemary oil* may boost hair growth, boost memory, prevent muscle spasms, and support the circulatory and nervous systems.

- *Sandalwood oil* is known by some to have aphrodisiac qualities.

- *Tea tree oil* is known to have antimicrobial, antiseptic, and disinfectant qualities. It is commonly found in shampoos and skincare products, to treat acne, burns, and bites. It works as mouth rinses, but it should never be swallowed, as it is harmful.

- *Thyme oil* is known to help reduce exhaustion, nervousness, and stress.

- *Yarrow oil* is used to treat symptoms of cold and flu, and also to reduce joint inflammation.

Essential oil for a therapeutic massage will be blended

with a "carrier oil" that dilutes the essential oil and lubrication.

Visiting an Aromatherapist

The aromatherapist should do a comprehensive health check; health background, lifestyle, diet, and current health status.

Aromatherapy involves a holistic strategy, so it seeks to treat a healthy person. Treatments will be based on the individual's physical and mental needs. Based on these needs, the aromatherapist may recommend a single essential oil or a mix. Based on the patient's needs and preferences, the practitioner may recommend a particular essential oil or a combination.

According to the National Cancer Institute (*NCI*), aromatherapy products don't need **FDA** approval as long as there is no proof that they treat a particular disease. An aromatherapist is different from a massage therapist, although a massage therapist could use aromatherapy oils.

Risks

Each oil has its chemical elements and the reason for its use, so it is important to consult with a trained aromatherapist, nurse, doctor, physical therapist, massage therapist, or pharmacist before applying or using essential oils for therapeutic purposes.

A certified professional can suggest and train interested persons on how to use each product, providing proper instructions on application or dilution. Consumers also need to remember that the U.S. Food and Drug Administration will not monitor aromatherapy products, so it might be challenging to know if a product is original or if it's contaminated or artificial.

Some beauty and home products, such as lotions, make-up, and candles, contain products that are essential oils; however, they are man-made fragrances.

Like drugs, essential oils must be treated with respect. It is essential to seek expert advice and to follow instructions carefully.

Caution when using essential oils

Since essential oils cause reactions in the body, not all oils will benefit everyone. Chemical substances in essential oils can produce unwanted effects when used with drugs. They could reduce the performance of everyday drugs, or they could exacerbate health issues in the average person.

A person with high blood pressure, for example, should avoid stimulants, such as rosemary. Some substances, such as fennel, aniseed, and sage, act like estrogen, so a person with an estrogen-dependent breast or ovarian tumor should avoid these.

Concentrated products may be poisonous before dilution and should be handled carefully. A maximum concentration of 5 percent is recommended. Some natural oils produce poisons that can damage the liver, kidneys, and nervous system, especially if swallowed. Swallowing essential oils can be dangerous and fatal in some cases.

People with the following conditions should be extra careful when working with aromatherapy:

- An allergy or allergies

- Hay fever, a kind of allergy

- Asthma

- Skin conditions such as eczema or psoriasis

People with the following conditions must be very careful:

- Epilepsy

- Hypertension or high blood pressure

If the oil is to be blended with a carrier, you should inform the aromatherapist or massage therapist about any nut allergies, because carrier oils tend to be extracted from nuts and seeds.

Aromatherapy can have diverse effects, but they are usually mild and don't last long.

They include:

- Nausea

- Headaches

- Other allergies

The use of aromatherapy by pregnant or nursing mothers is not proven safe by research so it is not recommended. During the first trimester of pregnancy, aromatherapy may pose a risk to the developing fetus. Women who are breastfeeding should avoid peppermint oil, as it might be obvious in breast milk.

Essential oils produced from citrus could make your skin sensitive to sunlight, increasing the chance of sunburn. Some natural oils may affect the function of everyday drugs, so people who are using any kind of drugs should speak with a professional pharmacist or doctor.

Finally, when storing essential oils, you must understand that light, heat, and oxygen affect the quality of the oil. Products should come from a known and reputable source to ensure product quality. Following instructions carefully reduces the potentials of harming the user's health.

In Elements of Traditional Western Europe, aromatherapy is integrated into mainstream medicine as an antiseptic, antiviral, antifungal, and antibacterial therapy. In America and Canada, this is also true. In France, some essential oils are used as prescription drugs, and they can only be given or recommended by a doctor. Aromatherapy can help treat some conditions, but it should be used correctly, under the supervision of a certified doctor. The **NAHA** can recommend aromatherapists locally, and some are members of a specialist association, however, there are no licensing boards for aromatherapists in the U.S.

Chapter 5

How Aromatherapy Works

When an essential oil is inhaled, the scent molecules enter the nasal cavity and stimulate the limbic system, a part of the brain that is important in emotion and behavior. The chemicals also stimulate the nervous system, which helps to regulate heartbeat, blood pressure, stress, inhaling, and exhaling. When used topically, the aroma chemicals are absorbed through the skin and inhaled.

The Study on Aromatherapy

As research on aromatherapy is somewhat limited, studies have researched the advantages of essential oils for several conditions. Here is a look at some results from the available proof:

- **Menstrual Pain**

Aromatherapy therapeutic massage over the stomach may help to cure menstrual pain, according to a written report published in Complementary Treatments in

Clinical Practice in 2017. Experts analyzed previously published clinical tests and discovered that aromatherapy therapeutic massage improved menstrual pain in comparison to therapeutic massage without aromatherapy.

- **Anxiety**

Inhaling the scent of an essential mix may reduce anxiety in women going through a breast biopsy. In a report published in Worldviews on Evidence-Based Medical, women received the lavender-sandalwood mix, an orange-peppermint blend, or a placebo. There is a reduction in anxiety by using the lavender-sandalwood blend.

- **Nausea**

Aromatherapy can reduce postoperative nausea and vomiting, according to a 2013 research published in Anesthesia and Analgesia. Experts discovered that nausea was reduced significantly after aromatherapy with ginger oil or a blend of essential oils of ginger, spearmint, peppermint, and cardamom. The use of essential oils was also associated with fewer demands for anti-nausea drugs.

- **Pain**

A report published in Complementary Therapies in Clinical Practice in 2016 evaluated the potency of lavender aromatherapy on depression, anxiety, and satisfaction in people getting an intravenous (IV) catheter before surgery. People used either lavender oil or a placebo. Following the process, pain and stress in those using lavender oil were reduced than in those who were found using the placebo. Satisfaction with the IV process was higher in people who used lavender oil.

Ways to use aromatherapy

Essential oils may also be used topically on the skin or inhaled:

- **Inhalation**

Essential oils can be put into a diffuser (*a tool that disperses the oils into the air*). There are various kinds of diffusers, including ceramic, reed, and ultrasonic diffusers. Jewelry diffusers, such as necklace and bracelet diffusers, are also available.

Topical Use

The most frequent topical use is in massage oil. Some people add a drop or two of essential oil to a warm shower. Essential oils can be bought in shampoo and skin products.

Side effects and safety

Essential oils can be poisonous when used internally. Also, a lot of people may experience irritation and contact dermatitis when they apply essential oils to the skin. A skin patch test should be carried out before using any new oil.

Essential oils shouldn't be applied in large quantities on the skin, or used in extreme quantities, or used for a long period of time. Besides skin discomfort and dermatitis, essential oils are absorbed through the skin and can be dangerous. Oils should be diluted with carrier oils. Pregnant and breastfeeding women and children should seek advice from their doctors before using essential oils.

You should learn more about how to use essential oils safely. If you are thinking of using aromatherapy for a disease, ensure to consult your doctor first to find out whether it suits you.

Chapter 6

Essential Oils and Diffusers: The Best Guide
4 Essential Oils for Rest & Relaxation

- **Lavender oil**

Lavender oil has been around for several years. The name is said to have originated from the Latin word "*lavare*," which means "to clean," or from the word "*livendulo*," which means "*livid or bluish*." It has been used worldwide for several different purposes and is one of the most popular essential oils today.

Although one of the most soothing essential oils; "*lavender*," has a variety of effects, in historical Egypt, it was often used for embalming and aesthetic purposes. In historic Rome, lavender was hyped because of its curing and antiseptic properties, and in the middle age, it was used throughout Britain to make furniture polish and also to make clothes smell good (*we still have lavender-scented laundry detergents today*).

Interesting fact! When the tomb of Ruler Tut was opened, several jars were discovered that included materials resembling lavender. This is a reminder that it was used as an embalming agent in ancient times.

Benefits & Results:

- Calming

- Lifts mood

- Alleviates panic and depression

- Anti-bacterial

- Anti-fungal

- Helps improve sleep

- Relieves PMS pain and tension

- Relieves headaches and migraines

Several tests have been carried out with lavender oil to prove its effectiveness in treating mental issues. One research showed that 60% of individuals who took lavender in supplementary form (*New Origins D-Stress*) noticed a 50% or even more reduction in their nervousness and depression symptoms, whereas only 43% of those going for a popular anti-depressant had the same results. It has been shown in studies to boost symptoms and issues related to **PTSD**, such as sleeplessness, mood swing, stress, and anxiety.

- **Chamomile oil**

Chamomile has been used therapeutically over several years, and as early as the first century for digestive issues. Like lavender, its uses are widespread across different parts of the world; however, many of its basic applications are cosmetics and also to soothe many different kinds of issues. It is a very gentle oil that is even ideal to be used on children.

There are two main types of chamomile:

Roman and German. *Roman chamomile* is indigenous to Western European countries and northern Africa but is currently harvested worldwide in various temperate areas. *German chamomile* is indigenous to European countries and Northwest Asia and still grows abundantly there to date.

Interesting fact! A reserve posting in 1911 called Plants Statements that chamomile has a great influence on other plants to keep them lively and energetic, and it is called the *"plant's doctor."* If it will keep plant life healthy, imagine what it can do for you!

Roman Chamomile oil

Benefits & Results:

- Soothing and calming

- Reduces anxiety and stress

- Good for headaches and migraines

- Reduces insomnia

- Anti-inflammatory

- Helps to relieve pain related to teething in infants

- One **controlled**, random clinical trial examined people who took chamomile pills to treat nervousness. The study showed that the procedure reduced stress symptoms in people who have moderate panic disorders.

- **Ylang OIL**

Ylang-ylang has a history of usefulness, but its medicinal properties weren't recognized until the early 20th century when it was used to treat many diseases like malaria, typhoid, and intestinal stress. Interestingly, it was also observed to have a positive influence on the heart when a condition arises – possibly the first indicator of its soothing abilities.

Ylang-ylang originates from the star-shaped plants of the ylang-ylang tree, mostly in Malaysia and some parts of East Asia and, today, Madaoilcar. The potency of ylang-ylang essential oils depends on when and the way the flowers of the tree are gathered.

Interesting fact! The ylang-ylang tree doesn't produce flowers until its fifth - twelve months of growth, but once it does, it produces around 45 pounds of blooms per year and can produce plants for up to 50 years.

Our favorite brand of this fragrance: **Aroma**

concentrated oils

Benefits & Results:

- Supports insomnia

- Suitable for high blood pressure

- Helps to calm, fast heartbeat

- Soothing and calming

- Good for nervousness and anxiety

- **Frankincense oil**

Frankincense has been valued and traded for up to 5,000 years and it is used in ceremonies or even to perfume temples, homes, and markets. It has always been acclaimed as a "heal-all" oil, used to treat from indigestion to coughs and colds to hemorrhoids. Today, we acknowledge the recovery and soothing benefits of this oil.

Frankincense oil comes from the Boswellia and Commiphora trees and shrubs. The bark of the trees and shrubs, when cut, produces a sap that thickens and is then steamed to make the frankincense oil.

Interesting fact! There were times when frankincense was worth more than platinum; the value of the product dropped when the Roman Empire fell, and trading routes were blocked.

Our favorite brand this aroma:

Now Essential oils

Now Frankincense oil

Benefits & Results:

- Calms anxiety
- Ease asthma
- Helps with colitis and Crohn's disease, and also cure other digestive disorders
- Relieves chronic stress

- Reduces pain and inflammation

- Boosts immunity

Four essential oils for higher concentration

- **ROSEMARY OIL**

You're probably familiar with using rosemary in your cooking, but how about in your diffuser? It was used extensively in ancient times for several purposes, including being used in marriages and for natural medicinal care.

Paracelsus, a renowned German-Swiss doctor, and botanist in the 16th century popularized rosemary oil and its ability to strengthen the whole body, and he specifically touted it due to its benefits to the liver, brain, and heart.

Interesting fact! Rosemary comes from the leaves of the seed, and in aromatherapy, the leaves are said to be the lungs of the plant, helping to supply air to the herb and strengthen it. In a nutshell, it provides it with life.

Our favorite brand of this fragrance: Pranarom Organic Oils

Rosemary Oil

Benefits & Results:

- Indigestion

- Digestive issues

- Detoxifying

- Revitalize thoughts

- Boost concentration

- Promote relaxed breathing

- **Cedarwood oil**

Cedarwood oil comes from a tree that is native to the United States and can grow up to about 1000 years. In historical Egypt, this oil was used in the mummification process, to repel bugs, and in makeup products.

Not only was cedarwood oil useful for concentration; in the last century, its positive effects on skin problems like eczema, and have been widely observed.

Interesting fact! Cedarwood oil is steam-distilled from the solid wood of the tree and also looks like yellow balsamic syrup. They have a warm, woody aroma.

Benefits & Results:

- Soothing
- Calming
- Diuretic
- Antispasmodic
- Antiseptic
- Fungicide
- Improves concentration
- Relieve spasms

- **Patchouli OIL**

Patchouli oil comes from a perennial herb that grows in Southeast Asia at heights between 3,000 and 6,000 ft. It was first used as a moth repellant and therefore was often used in the production of clothes.

Patchouli oil has improved with age – the old one is more desired when compared with the new one. It is regarded as a great balancer and helps to supply calm energy that allows many people to concentrate more and pay attention.

Interesting fact! Over time, patchouli oil has managed to lose the unpleasant smell that makes most people despise it and a sweeter aroma has now evolved. The natural oil has also changed from a light yellow to deep amber with time.

Benefits & Results:

- Reduces tension

- Good for meditation

- Relieves worries and stress

- Increases concentration

Skin applications - support lines and wrinkles, scars, and blemishes.

- **Eucalyptus oil**

The eucalyptus tree has so many benefits, it is believed that the oil of the tree might be antiseptic. The essential oil was initially distilled in the past in the 1700s for reducing chest colds, and many more uses of the oil were discovered in later years. More than 300 species and 700 types of eucalyptus and the trees have large root systems that absorb plenty of water, which resulted in it being planted in marshy, malaria-infested areas in an attempt to dry and purify the soil and air.

Interesting fact! The eucalyptus tree is one of the fastest-growing trees and shrubs in the world, reaching up to 480 feet. The oil has a long history of use, including its use during the first World War to regulate meningitis and flu outbreaks.

Benefits & Results:

- Natural insect repellant

- Decongestant

- Relieves muscle pains and aches

- Good for shingles

- Purifies air

- Improves concentration

- Antibacterial

Our favorite brand of this Aroma: Aromaforce Organic Oils

Eucalyptus oil

Four natural oils for emotion & happiness

- **Ruby Grapefruit oil**

Grapefruit, which was originally harvested in Asia, is currently harvested around the world in places like

America and Brazil. The fruit comes from a glossy-leaved tree that grows up to about 10 meters high. The oil from the grapefruit comes from the glands found deep in the peel of the fruit, which produces a small quantity of fat when pressed. The essential oil has a clean refreshing smell, and it is usually in pale yellow or light ruby color.

Interesting fact! Grapefruit oil is also from the citrus oil family, and therefore, should be used within six months of purchase.

Benefits & Results:

- Revives the brain

- Stimulates digestion

- Clears congestion

- Lifts mood

- Energizes.

- Invigorating.

- Encourages creativity

- Encourages playfulness

- An overall sense of happiness

- **Lemon Verbena oil**

This oil comes from the lemon verbena plant that was originally native to South U.S.A but was introduced in the 17th century to Europe. From the 18th century, it became known in the Mediterranean and some parts of the United States.

The lemon verbena flower has a thin stem and long, pale green leaves which pass through steam distillation to extract the oil. Lemon verbena oil has a fresh, lemony, sweet fragrance, and a pale olive or yellow color.

Interesting fact! Pure lemon verbena oil is sometimes difficult to find because often, sellers offer lemongrass oil or lemon balm oil, which is not like the pure lemon verbena oil.

Benefits & Results:

- Stimulates immunity

- Nourishes creativity

- Uplifting and invigorating

- Encourages imagination

- Promotes a happy mood

- Relieves nervousness and depression

- Cures respiratory problems

- **Bergamot OIL**

The bergamot tree has an evergreen origin, and it is thought to be a plant species between an orange tree and a citrus tree. Where the plant originally originated from is still being debated, from Southeast Asia to Europe to Greece; however, the oil is used as an antidote when people are under pressure, stress, or having mood swings. This oil is from the peel of the fruit of the bergamot tree when the fruit is pressed. Due to its citrus but spicy aroma, natural medicinal in perfumes, and other aesthetic applications.

Interesting fact! One of the most popular uses of bergamot is dark tea, which blends well to produce the favorite and popular Earl Gray tea.

Benefits & Results:

- Useful for respiratory system problems

- Treats skin issues

- Antiseptic

- Energizes

- Stimulates

- Relieves stress and tension

- **Orange oil**

Orange oil has perhaps one of the most extensive uses for essential oil, including being used for cooking, for aesthetic and cosmetics, as an air freshener or deodorant, and many more. For aromatherapy, though, it is acclaimed as a refreshing aroma with anti-depressant qualities. The oil is pressed from the peels of the oranges, just like other citrus oils.

Interesting fact! Orange oil has a distinctive quality of enhancing the secretion of glands, therefore, it has historically been used to enhance things like menstruation, lactation, and circulation of digestive juices or bile.

Benefits & Results:

- Settles digestive distress

- Invigorates

- Energizes

- Anti-Inflammatory

- Antiseptic

- Aphrodisiac

- Encourages positive feelings

Warm and Steam Oil Diffusers: How to Use Them

Now that we know what a few of the various essential oils are used for, how do we use them? Essential natural oils have a variety of uses and purposes including the therapeutic benefits we mentioned earlier; the best way to maximize all they have to offer is through aromatherapy. In today's world, this is simpler with the production of essential oil diffusers that help you to enjoy the numerous benefits and satisfactions of aromatherapy easily and without stress.

Concerning diffusers, there are two main types: *heat* and *steam*. If you're not familiar with essential oils or you want to consider your options, you must find out about the pros and cons of both types of diffusers to enable you to make the right choice.

Let's first take a look at *heat diffusers*. They are usually the cheapest option when it comes to diffusers. They have a reputation of being noiseless, and that implies that you won't even notice while it's diffusing the oils. Not all warm diffusers are made the same way; however, the best ones will produce low heat and more pleasant aromas. However, some high-temperature diffusers use high degrees of warmth to produce more powerful smells, but this may alter the chemical elements of the essential oil.

All heat diffusers have one major disadvantage: they have the possibility of dividing the essential oil into its different components because of the high temperature it uses. This implies that the entire essential oil won't enter the **environment,** because the oil has been divided and you won't get the same healing effects from the oil, which basically contradicts the goal of diffusing the natural essential oil for aromatherapy. However, you will still need to diffuse the natural oils for a pleasant smell in the environment.

Steam diffusers, on the other hand, do not require any kind of heat. Rather, it uses jets of air to draw the natural oil from beneath to the pipe and dispel them in a mist.

This sort of diffusion allows the entire essential oil to be dispersed into the air using small droplets. The essential oil does not break in any way or divide into different components which implies that you will be able to fully maximize the oil. When it comes to getting the best out of the benefits of aromatherapy, this is the best method.

While the machine is at work, there might be a little humming which is a result of the powerful work it is doing to quickly saturate the environment with the fragrance of the essential oil and the benefits you need.

Steam diffusers have one major disadvantage, they are usually more expensive than heat diffusers. However, if you want to enjoy the benefits of aromatherapy maximize the amount you spent in getting the natural essential oils, you should use a diffuser that won't damage or divide the natural oils. You should also use a diffuser that maximizes all of the natural oils and gives you your money's worth, while at the same allows you to enjoy their health benefits and beautiful fragrance. It is like buying a new Tv, you won't buy one that looks great but can't produce either sound or images. If you want to get the utmost satisfaction from natural oils then you should use the right equipment for diffusion.

When you're using diffusers, dilute the oil you want to use in a few glasses of water and turn the diffuser on. You can blend different oils together to producing a pleasing scent, though we'd advise that you ensure that you are only mixing natural oils that have the same therapeutic benefits. For instance, don't blend a relaxing essential oil with an energizing one if you wish to get relaxation benefits from the aromatherapy. There are several great blends you can get online with specific natural oils, and also plenty of pre-made mixes are available here or online!

Chapter 7

The Ultimate Essential Oil Guide: the ones to use and for what purpose

The world of essential oils is vast, intriguing, and honestly, a little bit confusing. Are these oils that powerful? (*Yes*). Do I have to be the Diy-loving, crunchy kind of person to use and enjoy them? Can I just dab a few drops on my skin daily? *(No, please don't)* How on earth can I maximize each of these different scents? *(We'll let you know!)*

To answer every essential oil-related FAQ, we enlisted the help of **Charlynn Avery**, aromatherapist and educator at **Aura Cacia**, to help us draft the best oil guide. Continue reading to get the knowledge on the best essential natural oils as well as how to use them.

What Are Essential Oils?

"Essential oils are highly concentrated, volatile seed extracts," explains Avery. "We get essential natural oils through a few different extraction methods, and the part of the plant we get the essential oil from can vary based on the essential oil but is usually the most aromatic part. Rose oil, for example, comes from the petals of the rose, while natural citrus oils come from the rind."

Because essential oils are all-natural, it might be easy to assume that they are gentle and usually unreactive. This is not in any way true-by description; it is potent stuff. *"Normally, they are up to 75 times stronger than dried herbs," says Avery*. Therefore, "essential oils must be handled carefully." This means that a few drops go a long way, and aside from specific oils (*more on that later*), essential oils should be diluted properly before applying them directly to the skin. Whether essential oils should be swallowed has become a highly debated topic, and many argue that it is not safe unless specifically recommended by a doctor or expert.

What can essential oils be used for?

Aromatherapy, treating skin conditions, soothing muscle irritation… the advantages of essential oils are numerous. "Essential oils can be used for personal care, in-home cleaning products, for general health in the context of emotional support, and several other ways," explains *Avery*. This flexibility also extends to the scents too. "A few of the most popular essential oils, like lavender and sweet orange, cross into many categories and can be used effectively for most applications," she says.

How should I dilute my natural oils?

Aside from avoiding a potential skin reaction, diluting essential oils also allows them to work better-when subjected to air alone; the molecules of the pure essential oils tend to evaporate rapidly. "Adding the essential oil to a carrier substance better facilitates the absorption of the oil by your body," *says Avery*.

Generally, (*even if you are adding the essential oils to a bath*), you may need a carrier oil-a natural, plant-based oil that can act as a base. Common carrier oils include sweet almond, jojoba, olive, sunflower seed, avocado, and grape seed.

According to Avery, while specific dilutions may differ

based on personal needs and individual essential oils, the general guideline is to aim for one percent to five percent dilution. "A one percent blend is six drops of oil per ounce of carrier, while a five percent blend would be 30 drops per ounce of carrier," she says.

Below, see which oils to use and how to sleep better, get rid of acne, headaches, and more.

- **TO FALL (AND STAY) ASLEEP:**

If you are counting sheep on a nightly basis, it might be high time for you to consider some aromatherapy. Countless studies give precise details on how beneficial certain scents can be in getting quality sleep, even in stressful situations. For instance, one study found that when **ICU** patients sniffed lavender, chamomile, and neroli, their anxiety levels dropped significantly, and their sleep quality did just the opposite. Another study found that the scent of lavender increased slow-wave (*deep*) sleep, especially in women. Just taking a whiff of any sleep-inducing oil before bed can help, but to reap the enormous benefits for as long as possible, consider keeping an open jar of the oil dilution on your nightstand or using a pillow spray.

Essential oils that help to induce sleep: lavender, vetiver, patchouli, sandalwood, ylang-ylang, chamomile, neroli, marjoram, cedar, bergamot, clary sage, frankincense, and rose.

- **FOR RELIEVING ANXIETY AND FINDING BALANCE:**

Don't panic; relaxation is a whiff away. While there are many science-backed scents for finding rest (*sandalwood, lavender, frankincense, and orange*), Avery highlights that in the long run, you need to do the following yourself: "Any aroma that speaks to you and brings a feeling of calm and relaxation can be beneficial." Well-known trick for alleviating tension in 30 seconds straight? Massage an oil blend with calming scents into your temples which are the pressure points.

Essential oils for relieving stress: rose, clary sage, frankincense, lavender, bergamot, marjoram, ylang-ylang, lemon, geranium, orange, sandalwood, chamomile, and vetiver.

- **For a mental boost**:

When the 4 p.m. clock strikes, reboot by sniffing an invigorating scent blend, or even better; spritz yourself with an oil-infused face mist. Take your pick of scents that will help you double down on the rest of the workday. One study shows that sniffing rosemary can increase memory by 75% while peppermint, also, has been associated with memory and sustained focus. Other research shows that peppermint, basil, and helichrysum help with burnout and mental fatigue.

Essential oils for boosting concentration: rosemary, basil, peppermint, helichrysum, cedar, vetiver, grapefruit, pine, juniper.

- **FOR INSTANT ENERGY:**

Skip the third cup of coffee and keep uplifting essential oils readily available instead. Citruses are explicitly known for improving mood and energy, alleviating fatigue-inducing anxiety, and stress. One study discovered that administering peppermint oil even resulted in a boost in exercise performance.

Essential oils for energy: lemon, orange, grapefruit, eucalyptus, cinnamon, peppermint, ginger, rosemary, spearmint, dark pepper, jasmine.

- **TO SOOTHE INFLAMMATION AND SKIN PROBLEM:**

We've discussed a lot about aiding mood and mentality, but how about the physical healing benefits of essential oils? Many plants are natural antiseptics, anti-inflammatories, antimicrobials, and antivirals, so when concentrated into oil form, they can act as effective remedies for acne, muscle soreness, sore throats, and more. Take ever-versatile peppermint oil, for example. "It's cooling, and its availability in formulated muscle care products alongside eucalyptus, wintergreen, and German chamomile essential oils to mention a few," Avery says: "Add ten drops of peppermint oil to 1 ounce of sweet almond oil, and rub it into leg muscles and feet."

As for blemishes and other skin irritations, there are many options as well. Tea tree oil is a preferred remedy for shriveling up zits in a matter of hours, especially since it is one of the only essential oils (*alongside lavender*) that can be safely applied directly on the skin. Dab a few drops on the blemish to zap bacteria and soothe any redness. Got irritated, inflamed skin from sunburn, rosacea, or other sensitivities? Mist on some rosewater or a lavender hydrosol for instant relief.

- **Essential oils for inflammation:**

- **Acne and skin irritations**: tea tree oil, lavender, oregano, bergamot, rosemary, helichrysum.

- **Muscle swelling:** peppermint, eucalyptus, wintergreen, chamomile, nutmeg, ginger, cayenne, rosemary, dark pepper.

- **Sore throat:** eucalyptus, peppermint, ginger, lemon, tea tree, sage, rosemary.

Chapter 8

Advantages and Disadvantages of Aromatherapy

Aromatherapy is an option in medicinal therapy where essential natural oils are inhaled to cure certain disorders such as stress and insomnia. And it's not new. Evidence shows its use on cave walls, historical writings, and Ruler Tut's tomb.

Because it has been around for several years, aromatherapy may be a highly effective treatment. However, in the eye of existing objectives, below are both the benefits and disadvantages of aromatherapy.

Advantages:

- **Healing Properties**

The primary benefits of aromatherapy are its known healing properties. Although there is little medical proof available today to aid its healing abilities. Medical professionals dating back to Hippocrates have touted its abilities. He, in truth, was known for thinking in *"vis medicatrix naturae,"* or "the curing power of character" and used aromatherapy as a staple in his curing practice.

Many general studies and reviews show evidence that aromatherapy with specific oils is incredibly useful for mood disorders, such as anxiety and depression.

- **Safe and natural**

While there are some exceptions, aromatherapy with essential oils is known to be safe and non-toxic for human inhalation. Essential oils are gotten from plants and if processed naturally, are organic substances. As a result of this, it's an exceptionally desirable option for man-made pharmaceuticals that have chemicals and substances foreign to nature. Using essential oils for aromatherapy, generally, will not harm humans, animals, or the environment.

- **Simplicity**

Aromatherapy is a relatively simple therapeutic process, with readily available products, and requires no professional supervision. The easiest method involves inhaling the product from its container, so there is no learning curve involved in treating yourself. And even in its most complicated form, you only will be adding one or more essential oils for some aromatherapy device, which may usually include instructions.

- **Availability**

Although aromatherapy has been around for years, its popularity has grown enormously in the last couple of years. As a result of this, oil companies are easy to find and access. There are lots of affordable products to fit almost any kind of budget.

Disadvantages:

- **Allergies**

Because oils are derived from plants, it stands to reason that people with a specific plant or seasonal allergy may be sensitive to certain essential oils. Allergic reactions are usually mild but should be taken into consideration when choosing your oils for aromatherapy.

- **Phototoxicity**

Citrus-based essential oils cause your skin to be sensitive to the sun's ultraviolet rays, sometimes causing deep sunburns. While basically, this is only an issue if applied directly to the skin. Safety measures should be taken after aromatherapy sessions using lemon, orange, grapefruit, or other citrus oils.

- **Lack of Medical Research**

Although some clinical studies are going on currently, there are many reasons you won't find much research on aromatherapy at the moment. Firstly, the essential oils aren't standardized. Because the elements of essential oils may differ based on harvest times, processes and climates, it's difficult to predict constant outcomes. Secondly, blind studies are difficult because fragrance is a major element of aromatherapy. And finally, since essential oils have been used on humans for years, there is no urgent need for testing as far as most government organizations are concerned. Rather than rely on the government for medical approval, you will have to learn from your errors and peer recommendations to making informed decisions.

- **Side Effects**

Because essential oils are usually safe and nontoxic, side effects are not common but should be taken into consideration, especially if certain medical conditions exist. Some possible side effects to know: headaches, nausea, rash, deep breathing difficulties (*in people with asthma*), and injury to a fetus. Usually, any side effect experienced from aromatherapy is a result of an already existing allergic condition. If you have known allergies, avoid essential oils gotten from those substances.

- **Flammable**

Essential oils are highly flammable and should not be used next to an open flame.

Is aromatherapy right for everybody?

While aromatherapy is relatively safe, there are a few

cases where aromatherapy and essential oils should be either avoided or used with extreme caution.

Pregnancy

Some natural oils are considered unsafe for pregnant women especially the following set of essential oils which are believed to cause instant miscarriage or contractions:

- Mugwort

- Parsley seed

- Pennyroyal

- Sage

- Sassafras

- Rue/Rutin

- Cottonwood Bark

- Tansy

- Wormwood

Studies were conducted on animals, and not humans; therefore, the level of precaution is a little uncertain and highly debated. Other essential oils such as *hyssop* are also considered questionable for use during pregnancy. It is considered best to avoid the use of all essential oils during pregnancy except under the care of a trained practitioner.

- **Hypertension**

Someone with hypertension should avoid stimulating essential oils such as rosemary, spike lavender, and cinnamon. These oils are used to stimulate blood circulation and energy.

- **Children**

Certain oils, such as *peppermint,* can be toxic to young children in high doses. While usually only harmful when applied topically, safety measures should be taken when used in aromatherapy as well.

- **Cancer**

Essential oils like fennel, sage, and clary sage contain

estrogen-like compounds. People with breasts or ovarian cancer should avoid such natural oils as they could feed the cancer cells. Always seek advice from your doctor and a certified aromatherapist before treating yourself with aromatherapy.

Chapter 9

How to use aromatherapy for stress relief

Aromatherapy has gained a lot of attention recently. Aromatherapy products, once relatively exotic, have finally sprung through to supermarkets shelves and aisles. Aromatherapy candles, shower products, essential oils, and other products are widely available and also have been acclaimed as helpful in calming babies, reducing stress, and promoting healthy living. But does aromatherapy surpass these claims?

Research

Relatively, there is little research on aromatherapy. While more studies are being conducted, it hasn't been "proven" like other stress relievers. However, while further studies are needed, many reports have previously shown the benefits of aromatherapy. Of the survey that is done today, below are some of the results:

1. Preliminary research demonstrates that aromatherapy can transform brain waves and

behavior.

2. Aromatherapy can reduce stress, increase contentment, and reduce cortisol levels, the "stress hormone."

3. Lavender aromatherapy has been proven to reduce crying in babies and enhance rest in newborns and adults.

4. Different aromatherapy scents produce different results in people. (*See this short article for aromatherapy: advantages of various smell*)

5. One research showed that aromatherapy therapeutic massage can have some beneficial effects on panic and depression.

6. Therapeutic massage with aromatherapy provides more powerful and more continuous rest from stress especially mental fatigue than therapeutic massage alone.

As a Stress Alleviation Tool

While aromatherapy isn't the magic 'cure-all' that it is sometimes made to look like, it has proven results as a stress reliever. Aromatherapy is a great tool for stress alleviation since it has a few (*if any*) known side effects, can be used passively (*you can cover the area with scent while you are engaged with other activities, alleviating stress along the way*), and can be easily used with other stress relievers (like therapeutic massage or yoga, for example), for increased stress comfort. Aromatherapy products are also accessible, making aromatherapy an easy option.

How to use aromatherapy for stress relieve

Aromatherapy is easy to use, specifically for busy people who need something quick. Below are a few ideas on how to use aromatherapy:

- **Candles**

Candles are great for aromatherapy. Lighting a candle is most likely one of the easiest ways to scent up a room and create a unique feeling, so get some good aromatherapy candles and let them burn. The candles, like incense, can also be used to create a relaxing atmosphere, or as a center point for deep breathing. However, they are more beneficial than some incense because they don't produce much smoke like cigarettes. Ensure you buy quality candles that give off an aroma that's powerful enough to be perceived around the area.

- **Diffusers**

Aromatherapy diffusers take essential oils and evaporate them into the environment. This is done using a candle or with batteries, if you would like to steer clear of open fire. Diffusers are excellent because they spread the aroma quite effectively. The battery-run ones can be safer than candles since no open fire is involved. This is another convenient way to create a soothing atmosphere, and look beautiful as well, increasing the calming vibe you can create at any time.

- **Body Products**

Aromatherapy body products are great because they produce a fragrance that follows you but can't necessarily be perceived by others (*unless they're very close, in which particular case they probably won't perceive*). You can rub aromatherapy cream over your skin, or dab a few drops of skincare essential oils on your veins and revel in the fragrance for hours.

Chapter 10

Six most popular new aromatherapy brands

1. Greenfrog Botanic

Based on the south coast in Hove, this beautiful new aromatherapy brand was made when **Nick Bridger**, an agricultural economist, met his new wife Julie, a French economist, working on human rights in Thailand. Then they relocated to India and discovered the country's soapberries, native to the Himalayas. For 'many monsoons', they experimented on berries and have now produced their first range.

They used a botanical soap from the Indian Himalayas, where it has been used for years in Hindu medicine for treating sensitive skin, then mix it with moisturizing organic aloe vera and aromatherapeutic essential oils, and then bottle it up. They're organic, Vegan qualified, cruelty-free, and contain zero parabens, palm oil, or Sodium Laureth Sulphate (*SLS*), and are produced in the United Kingdom.

Must have product: Botanical Bodywash

Coming in two completely different scents, this "mood-changing body wash" is the only shower gel you'll need. Neroli and Lime are ideal for your morning shower. They are energizing, zesty, and refreshing. There's also Peppermint and geranium; this is chilling, relaxing, and soothing. Using this at night helped me unwind and pull the plug, and I got into bed half as hyped up as I normally am. Might I add that they make you smell nice?

2. **1001 Remedies**

Having a mission statement of "Stand up to wellness," 1001 Remedies is a perfect choice for any Zen woman who lives by a clean-living mantra. Crafted by Parisian Sofia Belcadi, it is based on ancestral aromatherapy blends. Featuring formulas passed on by her Moroccan family of healers and apothecaries, the brand embodies the family's enthusiasm for curing and improving wellbeing. Sofia only uses 100 % natural ingredients, believing that plants preserve our local environment, empower the body, and reinforce our natural defenses. 1001 Remedies consists of five essential everyday products that provide therapeutic and effective solutions to your daily needs by working with your own natural defenses: and air spray, a face, body, and hair gel, a wrist balm to help promote, and two skincare products.

Must have product: PurAir Air Purifying spray

Made of 19 essential oils, including ravinstara, peppermint, and ho-wood, this addictive air-purifying spray is a handbag essential. It is ideal for your desk, at home, or on the go. It's a great antidote to combat environmental pollution and reinforce your natural defences. Together with everything, it smells divine; I can't remember what the office smells like before this. It's relaxing and calming but also made me alert.

3. **Puressentiel**

This well-loved French brand has finally been launched in the UK *(so basically new to us)*, bringing with them the Parisian love for aromatherapy and its health and well-being benefits. Produced by **Isabelle and Marco Pacchioni**, who shared a passion for aromatherapy and natural products, Puressentiel is an independent family company. By enlisting the help of botanists, experts, and doctors, they created a variety of products with essential oils and organic elements.

What makes Puressentiel so excellent is that they make aromatherapy accessible to everyone. They make complicated products that treat real illnesses but have amazing textures and scents, so you won't smell like a doctor's office.

Must have product - Puressentiel Bones Roller with 14 Essential Oils

The Muscle and Joint parts Roller is ideal for muscles before and after exercise as it relaxes and soothes. Made from 14 essential oils, including peppermint, rosemary, and chamomile, it's the perfect antidote to a strained muscle or stiff neck. I tried it on my neck after a long day of hunching over my laptop and felt better immediately. The smell was strong but comforting, and I couldn't stop rolling it all over my body.

4. Neom Organics

Neom was produced by **Nicola Elliott,** a trained aromatherapist and ex-magazine journalist who grew sick and tired of the continuous stress of 60 hours a week. Nicola believes that pure essential oils can help the well-being of women who face the pressure of modern day living, inadequate rest, high pressure, low energy, and mood. Recently, Neom has just dropped the most amazing collection yet, the scent to boost your energy range. Using complex blends of energizing essential oils such as grapefruit, Sicilian lemon, and cedarwood, they guarantee to enhance your energy every day.

Must have product - Feel Refreshed Reed Diffuser

The Feel Refreshed fragrance is a complex blend of 21 organic essential oils, including lemon and basil, with the sole purpose to stimulate a tired and busy mind and also encourage clear thinking. The diffuser fills the room with the beautiful smell, and it is the thing only thing you need on a Monday morning, humpday slump, or Friday evening lull (*so really all week*). The Feel Refreshed perfume can be bought as a candle, pillow mist, and home scent, which can help boost the immune system and kill bacteria in the air.

5. **Aroma Naturals**

Made by former pig-farmer **Diane Viall**, Aroma naturals are organic, handmade, and paraben, also **SLS** free. Diane started making her natural soaps and body oils as gifts for family and friends. Diane credits her hairdresser for getting the ball going, saying she was astonished at her homemade hair shampoo and asked Diane to make products for her to use and sell. Inspired by seeing her mum use witch hazel, olive oil, and lavender oil in homemade remedies, Diane even runs soap-making workshops from her farmhouse in North Norfolk.

Must have product - Oil candle

Her latest project is a new selection of luxury, hands poured, and natural candles. They burn for at least 40 hours and are ideal for a girl with a busy life because they are an ideal de-stress tool. I tried the simplicity candle on a particularly droopy Monday night and sensed my angst melting away with the wick. It is made from pure essential oils and soya wax and has been specially created to ensure you have the perfect beauty sleep.

6. **Olverum Bath Essential oil**

We're bending the rules slightly here as this is actually the same time-honoured formula since *Olverums'* inception in 1931, but it's too good, so we have a reason to talk about it. However, this bliss-inducing bath oil has been re-packaged, re-branded, and re-launched for all we modern aromatherapy advocates. It contains essential oils such as lemon, lavender, and exotic verbena, and you can even use it as a therapeutic massage oil and body moisturizer.

I put a few drops in my bath on a day where everything had gone wrong. My feet hurt, my nose was blocked, and my head was pounding. My dingy bathroom was suddenly transformed into a spa, and I re-emerged (*a good hour later*), I felt so calm, so I fell asleep right away.

The smell is unisex rather than too floral, which

makes it the sexiest-smelling bath oil around.

Choosing a Provider

You may wish to discuss with a qualified aromatherapist, especially when you're getting started with aromatherapy for the first time or if you have specific issues you'd like to discuss. You'll find an aromatherapist by using an online directory. Or ask at a spa or yoga studio.

While consulting with an aromatherapist, you'll answer questions and discuss your lifestyle and health. Together, you will come up with a personal treatment plan to meet your targets and manage your symptoms. You might have a few sessions with your aromatherapist, or you could choose to have continuous sessions for a longer time.

Since aromatherapy is a complementary therapy, you should speak with your doctor before starting your sessions. That way, your essential oil therapy can be tailored to work with any medical care or treatment you're receiving.

There are lots of information available online and in

books if you want to treat yourself at home. There are also courses you can take to learn more about aromatherapy.

Consultations with an aromatherapist will vary based on several factors, which include your location. You will probably pay up to $100 for a short consultation or up to $50 for follow-up consultations.